BLOOD PRESSURE LOG

NAME. ____

Date	AM		PM		Notes
	Blood pressure	Pulse	Blood pressure	Pulse	

Level of Severity	Systolic	Diastolic
Normal	120	80
Mild Hypertension	140-160	90-100
Moderate Hypertension	160-200	100-120
Severe Hypertension	Above 200	160-200

BLOOD PRESSURE LOG

NAME. ____

Date	AM		PM		Notes
	Blood pressure	Pulse	Blood pressure	Pulse	

Level of Severity	Systolic	Diastolic
Normal	120	80
Mild Hypertension	140-160	90-100
Moderate Hypertension	160-200	100-120
Severe Hypertension	Above 200	160-200

Blood Pressure Log

Name. ____

Date	AM		PM		Notes
	Blood pressure	Pulse	Blood pressure	Pulse	

Level of Severity	Systolic	Diastolic
Normal	120	80
Mild Hypertension	140-160	90-100
Moderate Hypertension	160-200	100-120
Severe Hypertension	Above 200	160-200

Blood Pressure Log

Name. ____

Date	AM		PM		Notes
	Blood pressure	Pulse	Blood pressure	Pulse	

Level of Severity	Systolic	Diastolic
Normal	120	80
Mild Hypertension	140-160	90-100
Moderate Hypertension	160-200	100-120
Severe Hypertension	Above 200	160-200

BLOOD PRESSURE LOG

NAME. _______________________________

Date	AM		PM		Notes
	Blood pressure	Pulse	Blood pressure	Pulse	

Level of Severity	Systolic	Diastolic
Normal	120	80
Mild Hypertension	140-160	90-100
Moderate Hypertension	160-200	100-120
Severe Hypertension	Above 200	160-200

BLOOD PRESSURE LOG

NAME. ____

Date	AM		PM		Notes
	Blood pressure	Pulse	Blood pressure	Pulse	

Level of Severity	Systolic	Diastolic
Normal	120	80
Mild Hypertension	140-160	90-100
Moderate Hypertension	160-200	100-120
Severe Hypertension	Above 200	160-200

Blood Pressure Log

NAME. ____

Date	AM		PM		Notes
	Blood pressure	Pulse	Blood pressure	Pulse	

Level of Severity	Systolic	Diastolic
Normal	120	80
Mild Hypertension	140-160	90-100
Moderate Hypertension	160-200	100-120
Severe Hypertension	Above 200	160-200

Blood Pressure Log

NAME. ____

Date	AM		PM		Notes
	Blood pressure	Pulse	Blood pressure	Pulse	

Level of Severity	Systolic	Diastolic
Normal	120	80
Mild Hypertension	140-160	90-100
Moderate Hypertension	160-200	100-120
Severe Hypertension	Above 200	160-200

Blood Pressure Log

Name. ____

Date	AM		PM		Notes
	Blood pressure	Pulse	Blood pressure	Pulse	

Level of Severity	Systolic	Diastolic
Normal	120	80
Mild Hypertension	140-160	90-100
Moderate Hypertension	160-200	100-120
Severe Hypertension	Above 200	160-200

BLOOD PRESSURE LOG

Name. ____

Date	AM		PM		Notes
	Blood pressure	Pulse	Blood pressure	Pulse	

Level of Severity	Systolic	Diastolic
Normal	120	80
Mild Hypertension	140-160	90-100
Moderate Hypertension	160-200	100-120
Severe Hypertension	Above 200	160-200

BLOOD PRESSURE LOG

NAME. ____

Date	AM		PM		Notes
	Blood pressure	Pulse	Blood pressure	Pulse	

Level of Severity	Systolic	Diastolic
Normal	120	80
Mild Hypertension	140-160	90-100
Moderate Hypertension	160-200	100-120
Severe Hypertension	Above 200	160-200

Blood Pressure Log

NAME. ____

Date	AM		PM		Notes
	Blood pressure	Pulse	Blood pressure	Pulse	

Level of Severity	Systolic	Diastolic
Normal	120	80
Mild Hypertension	140-160	90-100
Moderate Hypertension	160-200	100-120
Severe Hypertension	Above 200	160-200

Blood Pressure Log

Name. ____

Date	AM		PM		Notes
	Blood pressure	Pulse	Blood pressure	Pulse	

Level of Severity	Systolic	Diastolic
Normal	120	80
Mild Hypertension	140-160	90-100
Moderate Hypertension	160-200	100-120
Severe Hypertension	Above 200	160-200

BLOOD PRESSURE LOG

NAME. ____

Date	AM		PM		Notes
	Blood pressure	Pulse	Blood pressure	Pulse	

Level of Severity	Systolic	Diastolic
Normal	120	80
Mild Hypertension	140-160	90-100
Moderate Hypertension	160-200	100-120
Severe Hypertension	Above 200	160-200

Blood Pressure Log

Name. ____

Date	AM		PM		Notes
	Blood pressure	Pulse	Blood pressure	Pulse	

Level of Severity	Systolic	Diastolic
Normal	120	80
Mild Hypertension	140-160	90-100
Moderate Hypertension	160-200	100-120
Severe Hypertension	Above 200	160-200

BLOOD PRESSURE LOG

NAME. ____

Date	AM		PM		Notes
	Blood pressure	Pulse	Blood pressure	Pulse	

Level of Severity	Systolic	Diastolic
Normal	120	80
Mild Hypertension	140-160	90-100
Moderate Hypertension	160-200	100-120
Severe Hypertension	Above 200	160-200

Blood Pressure Log

NAME. ____

Date	AM		PM		Notes
	Blood pressure	Pulse	Blood pressure	Pulse	

Level of Severity	Systolic	Diastolic
Normal	120	80
Mild Hypertension	140-160	90-100
Moderate Hypertension	160-200	100-120
Severe Hypertension	Above 200	160-200

BLOOD PRESSURE LOG

NAME. _______________________________

Date	AM		PM		Notes
	Blood pressure	Pulse	Blood pressure	Pulse	

Level of Severity	Systolic	Diastolic
Normal	120	80
Mild Hypertension	140-160	90-100
Moderate Hypertension	160-200	100-120
Severe Hypertension	Above 200	160-200

Blood Pressure Log

NAME. ____

Date	AM		PM		Notes
	Blood pressure	Pulse	Blood pressure	Pulse	

Level of Severity	Systolic	Diastolic
Normal	120	80
Mild Hypertension	140-160	90-100
Moderate Hypertension	160-200	100-120
Severe Hypertension	Above 200	160-200

Blood Pressure Log

NAME. ____

Date	AM		PM		Notes
	Blood pressure	Pulse	Blood pressure	Pulse	

Level of Severity	Systolic	Diastolic
Normal	120	80
Mild Hypertension	140-160	90-100
Moderate Hypertension	160-200	100-120
Severe Hypertension	Above 200	160-200

Blood Pressure Log

NAME. ____

Date	AM		PM		Notes
	Blood pressure	Pulse	Blood pressure	Pulse	

Level of Severity	Systolic	Diastolic
Normal	120	80
Mild Hypertension	140-160	90-100
Moderate Hypertension	160-200	100-120
Severe Hypertension	Above 200	160-200

Blood Pressure Log

NAME. ____

Date	AM		PM		Notes
	Blood pressure	Pulse	Blood pressure	Pulse	

Level of Severity	Systolic	Diastolic
Normal	120	80
Mild Hypertension	140-160	90-100
Moderate Hypertension	160-200	100-120
Severe Hypertension	Above 200	160-200

Blood Pressure Log

NAME. ____

Date	AM		PM		Notes
	Blood pressure	Pulse	Blood pressure	Pulse	

Level of Severity	Systolic	Diastolic
Normal	120	80
Mild Hypertension	140-160	90-100
Moderate Hypertension	160-200	100-120
Severe Hypertension	Above 200	160-200

Blood Pressure Log

Name. ____

Date	AM		PM		Notes
	Blood pressure	Pulse	Blood pressure	Pulse	

Level of Severity	Systolic	Diastolic
Normal	120	80
Mild Hypertension	140-160	90-100
Moderate Hypertension	160-200	100-120
Severe Hypertension	Above 200	160-200

Blood Pressure Log

Name. ____

Date	AM		PM		Notes
	Blood pressure	Pulse	Blood pressure	Pulse	

Level of Severity	Systolic	Diastolic
Normal	120	80
Mild Hypertension	140-160	90-100
Moderate Hypertension	160-200	100-120
Severe Hypertension	Above 200	160-200

BLOOD PRESSURE LOG

NAME. ____

Date	AM		PM		Notes
	Blood pressure	Pulse	Blood pressure	Pulse	

Level of Severity	Systolic	Diastolic
Normal	120	80
Mild Hypertension	140-160	90-100
Moderate Hypertension	160-200	100-120
Severe Hypertension	Above 200	160-200

BLOOD PRESSURE LOG

NAME. ____

Date	AM		PM		Notes
	Blood pressure	Pulse	Blood pressure	Pulse	

Level of Severity	Systolic	Diastolic
Normal	120	80
Mild Hypertension	140-160	90-100
Moderate Hypertension	160-200	100-120
Severe Hypertension	Above 200	160-200

BLOOD PRESSURE LOG

NAME. ____

Date	AM		PM		Notes
	Blood pressure	Pulse	Blood pressure	Pulse	

Level of Severity	Systolic	Diastolic
Normal	120	80
Mild Hypertension	140-160	90-100
Moderate Hypertension	160-200	100-120
Severe Hypertension	Above 200	160-200

Blood Pressure Log

Name. ____

Date	AM		PM		Notes
	Blood pressure	Pulse	Blood pressure	Pulse	

Level of Severity	Systolic	Diastolic
Normal	120	80
Mild Hypertension	140-160	90-100
Moderate Hypertension	160-200	100-120
Severe Hypertension	Above 200	160-200

Blood Pressure Log

NAME. ____

Date	AM		PM		Notes
	Blood pressure	Pulse	Blood pressure	Pulse	

Level of Severity	Systolic	Diastolic
Normal	120	80
Mild Hypertension	140-160	90-100
Moderate Hypertension	160-200	100-120
Severe Hypertension	Above 200	160-200

BLOOD PRESSURE LOG

NAME. ____

Date	AM		PM		Notes
	Blood pressure	Pulse	Blood pressure	Pulse	

Level of Severity	Systolic	Diastolic
Normal	120	80
Mild Hypertension	140-160	90-100
Moderate Hypertension	160-200	100-120
Severe Hypertension	Above 200	160-200

BLOOD PRESSURE LOG

NAME. ____

Date	AM		PM		Notes
	Blood pressure	Pulse	Blood pressure	Pulse	

Level of Severity	Systolic	Diastolic
Normal	120	80
Mild Hypertension	140-160	90-100
Moderate Hypertension	160-200	100-120
Severe Hypertension	Above 200	160-200

Blood Pressure Log

NAME. ____

Date	AM		PM		Notes
	Blood pressure	Pulse	Blood pressure	Pulse	

Level of Severity	Systolic	Diastolic
Normal	120	80
Mild Hypertension	140-160	90-100
Moderate Hypertension	160-200	100-120
Severe Hypertension	Above 200	160-200

BLOOD PRESSURE LOG

NAME. ____

Date	AM		PM		Notes
	Blood pressure	Pulse	Blood pressure	Pulse	

Level of Severity	Systolic	Diastolic
Normal	120	80
Mild Hypertension	140-160	90-100
Moderate Hypertension	160-200	100-120
Severe Hypertension	Above 200	160-200

BLOOD PRESSURE LOG

NAME. ____

Date	AM		PM		Notes
	Blood pressure	Pulse	Blood pressure	Pulse	

Level of Severity	Systolic	Diastolic
Normal	120	80
Mild Hypertension	140-160	90-100
Moderate Hypertension	160-200	100-120
Severe Hypertension	Above 200	160-200

Blood Pressure Log

Name. ____

| Date | AM | | PM | | Notes |
	Blood pressure	Pulse	Blood pressure	Pulse	

Level of Severity	Systolic	Diastolic
Normal	120	80
Mild Hypertension	140-160	90-100
Moderate Hypertension	160-200	100-120
Severe Hypertension	Above 200	160-200

Blood Pressure Log

Name. ____

Date	AM		PM		Notes
	Blood pressure	Pulse	Blood pressure	Pulse	

Level of Severity	Systolic	Diastolic
Normal	120	80
Mild Hypertension	140-160	90-100
Moderate Hypertension	160-200	100-120
Severe Hypertension	Above 200	160-200

Blood Pressure Log

Name. ____

Date	AM		PM		Notes
	Blood pressure	Pulse	Blood pressure	Pulse	

Level of Severity	Systolic	Diastolic
Normal	120	80
Mild Hypertension	140-160	90-100
Moderate Hypertension	160-200	100-120
Severe Hypertension	Above 200	160-200

Blood Pressure Log

NAME. ____

Date	AM		PM		Notes
	Blood pressure	Pulse	Blood pressure	Pulse	

Level of Severity	Systolic	Diastolic
Normal	120	80
Mild Hypertension	140-160	90-100
Moderate Hypertension	160-200	100-120
Severe Hypertension	Above 200	160-200

BLOOD PRESSURE LOG

NAME. ____

Date	AM		PM		Notes
	Blood pressure	Pulse	Blood pressure	Pulse	

Level of Severity	Systolic	Diastolic
Normal	120	80
Mild Hypertension	140-160	90-100
Moderate Hypertension	160-200	100-120
Severe Hypertension	Above 200	160-200

BLOOD PRESSURE LOG

NAME. ____

Date	AM		PM		Notes
	Blood pressure	Pulse	Blood pressure	Pulse	

Level of Severity	Systolic	Diastolic
Normal	120	80
Mild Hypertension	140-160	90-100
Moderate Hypertension	160-200	100-120
Severe Hypertension	Above 200	160-200

BLOOD PRESSURE LOG

NAME. ____

Date	AM		PM		Notes
	Blood pressure	Pulse	Blood pressure	Pulse	

Level of Severity	Systolic	Diastolic
Normal	120	80
Mild Hypertension	140-160	90-100
Moderate Hypertension	160-200	100-120
Severe Hypertension	Above 200	160-200

BLOOD PRESSURE LOG

NAME. ____

| Date | AM | | PM | | Notes |
	Blood pressure	Pulse	Blood pressure	Pulse	

Level of Severity	Systolic	Diastolic
Normal	120	80
Mild Hypertension	140-160	90-100
Moderate Hypertension	160-200	100-120
Severe Hypertension	Above 200	160-200

BLOOD PRESSURE LOG

NAME. ____

Date	AM		PM		Notes
	Blood pressure	Pulse	Blood pressure	Pulse	

Level of Severity	Systolic	Diastolic
Normal	120	80
Mild Hypertension	140-160	90-100
Moderate Hypertension	160-200	100-120
Severe Hypertension	Above 200	160-200

BLOOD PRESSURE LOG

NAME. ____

| Date | AM | | PM | | Notes |
	Blood pressure	Pulse	Blood pressure	Pulse	

Level of Severity	Systolic	Diastolic
Normal	120	80
Mild Hypertension	140-160	90-100
Moderate Hypertension	160-200	100-120
Severe Hypertension	Above 200	160-200

BLOOD PRESSURE LOG

NAME. ____

Date	AM		PM		Notes
	Blood pressure	Pulse	Blood pressure	Pulse	

Level of Severity	Systolic	Diastolic
Normal	120	80
Mild Hypertension	140-160	90-100
Moderate Hypertension	160-200	100-120
Severe Hypertension	Above 200	160-200

BLOOD PRESSURE LOG

NAME. _______________________________

Date	AM		PM		Notes
	Blood pressure	Pulse	Blood pressure	Pulse	

Level of Severity	Systolic	Diastolic
Normal	120	80
Mild Hypertension	140-160	90-100
Moderate Hypertension	160-200	100-120
Severe Hypertension	Above 200	160-200

BLOOD PRESSURE LOG

NAME. ____

Date	AM		PM		Notes
	Blood pressure	Pulse	Blood pressure	Pulse	

Level of Severity	Systolic	Diastolic
Normal	120	80
Mild Hypertension	140-160	90-100
Moderate Hypertension	160-200	100-120
Severe Hypertension	Above 200	160-200

Blood Pressure Log

Name. ____

Date	AM		PM		Notes
	Blood pressure	Pulse	Blood pressure	Pulse	

Level of Severity	Systolic	Diastolic
Normal	120	80
Mild Hypertension	140-160	90-100
Moderate Hypertension	160-200	100-120
Severe Hypertension	Above 200	160-200

Blood Pressure Log

NAME. _______________________________

Date	AM		PM		Notes
	Blood pressure	Pulse	Blood pressure	Pulse	

Level of Severity	Systolic	Diastolic
Normal	120	80
Mild Hypertension	140-160	90-100
Moderate Hypertension	160-200	100-120
Severe Hypertension	Above 200	160-200

BLOOD PRESSURE LOG

NAME. ____

Date	AM		PM		Notes
	Blood pressure	Pulse	Blood pressure	Pulse	

Level of Severity	Systolic	Diastolic
Normal	120	80
Mild Hypertension	140-160	90-100
Moderate Hypertension	160-200	100-120
Severe Hypertension	Above 200	160-200

Blood Pressure Log

Name. ___________________________________

Date	AM		PM		Notes
	Blood pressure	Pulse	Blood pressure	Pulse	

Level of Severity	Systolic	Diastolic
Normal	120	80
Mild Hypertension	140-160	90-100
Moderate Hypertension	160-200	100-120
Severe Hypertension	Above 200	160-200

Blood Pressure Log

Name. ____

Date	AM		PM		Notes
	Blood pressure	Pulse	Blood pressure	Pulse	

Level of Severity	Systolic	Diastolic
Normal	120	80
Mild Hypertension	140-160	90-100
Moderate Hypertension	160-200	100-120
Severe Hypertension	Above 200	160-200

BLOOD PRESSURE LOG

NAME. ____

Date	AM		PM		Notes
	Blood pressure	Pulse	Blood pressure	Pulse	

Level of Severity	Systolic	Diastolic
Normal	120	80
Mild Hypertension	140-160	90-100
Moderate Hypertension	160-200	100-120
Severe Hypertension	Above 200	160-200

BLOOD PRESSURE LOG

NAME. ____

| Date | AM | | PM | | Notes |
	Blood pressure	Pulse	Blood pressure	Pulse	

Level of Severity	Systolic	Diastolic
Normal	120	80
Mild Hypertension	140-160	90-100
Moderate Hypertension	160-200	100-120
Severe Hypertension	Above 200	160-200

Blood Pressure Log

Name. ____

Date	AM		PM		Notes
	Blood pressure	Pulse	Blood pressure	Pulse	

Level of Severity	Systolic	Diastolic
Normal	120	80
Mild Hypertension	140-160	90-100
Moderate Hypertension	160-200	100-120
Severe Hypertension	Above 200	160-200

Blood Pressure Log

Name. ____

Date	AM		PM		Notes
	Blood pressure	Pulse	Blood pressure	Pulse	

Level of Severity	Systolic	Diastolic
Normal	120	80
Mild Hypertension	140-160	90-100
Moderate Hypertension	160-200	100-120
Severe Hypertension	Above 200	160-200

Blood Pressure Log

NAME. ____

Date	AM		PM		Notes
	Blood pressure	Pulse	Blood pressure	Pulse	

Level of Severity	Systolic	Diastolic
Normal	120	80
Mild Hypertension	140-160	90-100
Moderate Hypertension	160-200	100-120
Severe Hypertension	Above 200	160-200

Blood Pressure Log

NAME. ____

Date	AM		PM		Notes
	Blood pressure	Pulse	Blood pressure	Pulse	

Level of Severity	Systolic	Diastolic
Normal	120	80
Mild Hypertension	140-160	90-100
Moderate Hypertension	160-200	100-120
Severe Hypertension	Above 200	160-200

BLOOD PRESSURE LOG

NAME. ____

Date	AM		PM		Notes
	Blood pressure	Pulse	Blood pressure	Pulse	

Level of Severity	Systolic	Diastolic
Normal	120	80
Mild Hypertension	140-160	90-100
Moderate Hypertension	160-200	100-120
Severe Hypertension	Above 200	160-200

BLOOD PRESSURE LOG

NAME. ____

Date	AM		PM		Notes
	Blood pressure	Pulse	Blood pressure	Pulse	

Level of Severity	Systolic	Diastolic
Normal	120	80
Mild Hypertension	140-160	90-100
Moderate Hypertension	160-200	100-120
Severe Hypertension	Above 200	160-200

Blood Pressure Log

Name. ____

Date	AM		PM		Notes
	Blood pressure	Pulse	Blood pressure	Pulse	

Level of Severity	Systolic	Diastolic
Normal	120	80
Mild Hypertension	140-160	90-100
Moderate Hypertension	160-200	100-120
Severe Hypertension	Above 200	160-200

BLOOD PRESSURE LOG

NAME. ____

Date	AM		PM		Notes
	Blood pressure	Pulse	Blood pressure	Pulse	

Level of Severity	Systolic	Diastolic
Normal	120	80
Mild Hypertension	140-160	90-100
Moderate Hypertension	160-200	100-120
Severe Hypertension	Above 200	160-200

BLOOD PRESSURE LOG

NAME. ____

Date	AM		PM		Notes
	Blood pressure	Pulse	Blood pressure	Pulse	

Level of Severity	Systolic	Diastolic
Normal	120	80
Mild Hypertension	140-160	90-100
Moderate Hypertension	160-200	100-120
Severe Hypertension	Above 200	160-200

BLOOD PRESSURE LOG

NAME. ____

Date	AM		PM		Notes
	Blood pressure	Pulse	Blood pressure	Pulse	

Level of Severity	Systolic	Diastolic
Normal	120	80
Mild Hypertension	140-160	90-100
Moderate Hypertension	160-200	100-120
Severe Hypertension	Above 200	160-200

BLOOD PRESSURE LOG

NAME. ____

Date	AM		PM		Notes
	Blood pressure	Pulse	Blood pressure	Pulse	

Level of Severity	Systolic	Diastolic
Normal	120	80
Mild Hypertension	140-160	90-100
Moderate Hypertension	160-200	100-120
Severe Hypertension	Above 200	160-200

BLOOD PRESSURE LOG

NAME. __________________________________

Date	AM		PM		Notes
	Blood pressure	Pulse	Blood pressure	Pulse	

Level of Severity	Systolic	Diastolic
Normal	120	80
Mild Hypertension	140-160	90-100
Moderate Hypertension	160-200	100-120
Severe Hypertension	Above 200	160-200

BLOOD PRESSURE LOG

NAME. ____

Date	AM		PM		Notes
	Blood pressure	Pulse	Blood pressure	Pulse	

Level of Severity	Systolic	Diastolic
Normal	120	80
Mild Hypertension	140-160	90-100
Moderate Hypertension	160-200	100-120
Severe Hypertension	Above 200	160-200

BLOOD PRESSURE LOG

NAME. ____

Date	AM		PM		Notes
	Blood pressure	Pulse	Blood pressure	Pulse	

Level of Severity	Systolic	Diastolic
Normal	120	80
Mild Hypertension	140-160	90-100
Moderate Hypertension	160-200	100-120
Severe Hypertension	Above 200	160-200

Blood Pressure Log

NAME. ____

Date	AM		PM		Notes
	Blood pressure	Pulse	Blood pressure	Pulse	

Level of Severity	Systolic	Diastolic
Normal	120	80
Mild Hypertension	140-160	90-100
Moderate Hypertension	160-200	100-120
Severe Hypertension	Above 200	160-200

BLOOD PRESSURE LOG

NAME. ____

Date	AM		PM		Notes
	Blood pressure	Pulse	Blood pressure	Pulse	

Level of Severity	Systolic	Diastolic
Normal	120	80
Mild Hypertension	140-160	90-100
Moderate Hypertension	160-200	100-120
Severe Hypertension	Above 200	160-200

BLOOD PRESSURE LOG

NAME. ____

Date	AM		PM		Notes
	Blood pressure	Pulse	Blood pressure	Pulse	

Level of Severity	Systolic	Diastolic
Normal	120	80
Mild Hypertension	140-160	90-100
Moderate Hypertension	160-200	100-120
Severe Hypertension	Above 200	160-200

BLOOD PRESSURE LOG

NAME. ____

Date	AM		PM		Notes
	Blood pressure	Pulse	Blood pressure	Pulse	

Level of Severity	Systolic	Diastolic
Normal	120	80
Mild Hypertension	140-160	90-100
Moderate Hypertension	160-200	100-120
Severe Hypertension	Above 200	160-200

BLOOD PRESSURE LOG

NAME. ____

Date	AM		PM		Notes
	Blood pressure	Pulse	Blood pressure	Pulse	

Level of Severity	Systolic	Diastolic
Normal	120	80
Mild Hypertension	140-160	90-100
Moderate Hypertension	160-200	100-120
Severe Hypertension	Above 200	160-200

BLOOD PRESSURE LOG

NAME. ____

Date	AM		PM		Notes
	Blood pressure	Pulse	Blood pressure	Pulse	

Level of Severity	Systolic	Diastolic
Normal	120	80
Mild Hypertension	140-160	90-100
Moderate Hypertension	160-200	100-120
Severe Hypertension	Above 200	160-200

Blood Pressure Log

Name. ____

Date	AM		PM		Notes
	Blood pressure	Pulse	Blood pressure	Pulse	

Level of Severity	Systolic	Diastolic
Normal	120	80
Mild Hypertension	140-160	90-100
Moderate Hypertension	160-200	100-120
Severe Hypertension	Above 200	160-200

BLOOD PRESSURE LOG

NAME. ____

Date	AM		PM		Notes
	Blood pressure	Pulse	Blood pressure	Pulse	

Level of Severity	Systolic	Diastolic
Normal	120	80
Mild Hypertension	140-160	90-100
Moderate Hypertension	160-200	100-120
Severe Hypertension	Above 200	160-200

BLOOD PRESSURE LOG

NAME. ____

Date	AM		PM		Notes
	Blood pressure	Pulse	Blood pressure	Pulse	

Level of Severity	Systolic	Diastolic
Normal	120	80
Mild Hypertension	140-160	90-100
Moderate Hypertension	160-200	100-120
Severe Hypertension	Above 200	160-200

Blood Pressure Log

Name. ____

Date	AM		PM		Notes
	Blood pressure	Pulse	Blood pressure	Pulse	

Level of Severity	Systolic	Diastolic
Normal	120	80
Mild Hypertension	140-160	90-100
Moderate Hypertension	160-200	100-120
Severe Hypertension	Above 200	160-200

BLOOD PRESSURE LOG

NAME. ____

Date	AM		PM		Notes
	Blood pressure	Pulse	Blood pressure	Pulse	

Level of Severity	Systolic	Diastolic
Normal	120	80
Mild Hypertension	140-160	90-100
Moderate Hypertension	160-200	100-120
Severe Hypertension	Above 200	160-200

Blood Pressure Log

Name. ____

Date	AM		PM		Notes
	Blood pressure	Pulse	Blood pressure	Pulse	

Level of Severity	Systolic	Diastolic
Normal	120	80
Mild Hypertension	140-160	90-100
Moderate Hypertension	160-200	100-120
Severe Hypertension	Above 200	160-200

BLOOD PRESSURE LOG

NAME. ____

Date	AM		PM		Notes
	Blood pressure	Pulse	Blood pressure	Pulse	

Level of Severity	Systolic	Diastolic
Normal	120	80
Mild Hypertension	140-160	90-100
Moderate Hypertension	160-200	100-120
Severe Hypertension	Above 200	160-200

BLOOD PRESSURE LOG

NAME. ____

Date	AM		PM		Notes
	Blood pressure	Pulse	Blood pressure	Pulse	

Level of Severity	Systolic	Diastolic
Normal	120	80
Mild Hypertension	140-160	90-100
Moderate Hypertension	160-200	100-120
Severe Hypertension	Above 200	160-200

BLOOD PRESSURE LOG

NAME. ____

Date	AM		PM		Notes
	Blood pressure	Pulse	Blood pressure	Pulse	

Level of Severity	Systolic	Diastolic
Normal	120	80
Mild Hypertension	140-160	90-100
Moderate Hypertension	160-200	100-120
Severe Hypertension	Above 200	160-200

BLOOD PRESSURE LOG

NAME. ____

Date	AM		PM		Notes
	Blood pressure	Pulse	Blood pressure	Pulse	

Level of Severity	Systolic	Diastolic
Normal	120	80
Mild Hypertension	140-160	90-100
Moderate Hypertension	160-200	100-120
Severe Hypertension	Above 200	160-200

BLOOD PRESSURE LOG

NAME. ____

Date	AM		PM		Notes
	Blood pressure	Pulse	Blood pressure	Pulse	

Level of Severity	Systolic	Diastolic
Normal	120	80
Mild Hypertension	140-160	90-100
Moderate Hypertension	160-200	100-120
Severe Hypertension	Above 200	160-200

BLOOD PRESSURE LOG

NAME. ____

Date	AM		PM		Notes
	Blood pressure	Pulse	Blood pressure	Pulse	

Level of Severity	Systolic	Diastolic
Normal	120	80
Mild Hypertension	140-160	90-100
Moderate Hypertension	160-200	100-120
Severe Hypertension	Above 200	160-200

BLOOD PRESSURE LOG

NAME. ____

Date	AM		PM		Notes
	Blood pressure	Pulse	Blood pressure	Pulse	

Level of Severity	Systolic	Diastolic
Normal	120	80
Mild Hypertension	140-160	90-100
Moderate Hypertension	160-200	100-120
Severe Hypertension	Above 200	160-200

BLOOD PRESSURE LOG

NAME. ____

Date	AM		PM		Notes
	Blood pressure	Pulse	Blood pressure	Pulse	

Level of Severity	Systolic	Diastolic
Normal	120	80
Mild Hypertension	140-160	90-100
Moderate Hypertension	160-200	100-120
Severe Hypertension	Above 200	160-200

BLOOD PRESSURE LOG

NAME. ____

Date	AM		PM		Notes
	Blood pressure	Pulse	Blood pressure	Pulse	

Level of Severity	Systolic	Diastolic
Normal	120	80
Mild Hypertension	140-160	90-100
Moderate Hypertension	160-200	100-120
Severe Hypertension	Above 200	160-200

Blood Pressure Log

Name. ____

Date	AM		PM		Notes
	Blood pressure	Pulse	Blood pressure	Pulse	

Level of Severity	Systolic	Diastolic
Normal	120	80
Mild Hypertension	140-160	90-100
Moderate Hypertension	160-200	100-120
Severe Hypertension	Above 200	160-200

Blood Pressure Log

Name. ____

Date	AM		PM		Notes
	Blood pressure	Pulse	Blood pressure	Pulse	

Level of Severity	Systolic	Diastolic
Normal	120	80
Mild Hypertension	140-160	90-100
Moderate Hypertension	160-200	100-120
Severe Hypertension	Above 200	160-200

Blood Pressure Log

NAME. ____

Date	AM		PM		Notes
	Blood pressure	Pulse	Blood pressure	Pulse	

Level of Severity	Systolic	Diastolic
Normal	120	80
Mild Hypertension	140-160	90-100
Moderate Hypertension	160-200	100-120
Severe Hypertension	Above 200	160-200

BLOOD PRESSURE LOG

NAME. ____

Date	AM		PM		Notes
	Blood pressure	Pulse	Blood pressure	Pulse	

Level of Severity	Systolic	Diastolic
Normal	120	80
Mild Hypertension	140-160	90-100
Moderate Hypertension	160-200	100-120
Severe Hypertension	Above 200	160-200

Blood Pressure Log

Name. _______________________________

Date	AM		PM		Notes
	Blood pressure	Pulse	Blood pressure	Pulse	

Level of Severity	Systolic	Diastolic
Normal	120	80
Mild Hypertension	140-160	90-100
Moderate Hypertension	160-200	100-120
Severe Hypertension	Above 200	160-200

BLOOD PRESSURE LOG

NAME. ____

Date	AM		PM		Notes
	Blood pressure	Pulse	Blood pressure	Pulse	

Level of Severity	Systolic	Diastolic
Normal	120	80
Mild Hypertension	140-160	90-100
Moderate Hypertension	160-200	100-120
Severe Hypertension	Above 200	160-200

Blood Pressure Log

NAME. ____

Date	AM		PM		Notes
	Blood pressure	Pulse	Blood pressure	Pulse	

Level of Severity	Systolic	Diastolic
Normal	120	80
Mild Hypertension	140-160	90-100
Moderate Hypertension	160-200	100-120
Severe Hypertension	Above 200	160-200

Blood Pressure Log

NAME. ____

Date	AM		PM		Notes
	Blood pressure	Pulse	Blood pressure	Pulse	

Level of Severity	Systolic	Diastolic
Normal	120	80
Mild Hypertension	140-160	90-100
Moderate Hypertension	160-200	100-120
Severe Hypertension	Above 200	160-200

BLOOD PRESSURE LOG

NAME. ____

Date	AM		PM		Notes
	Blood pressure	Pulse	Blood pressure	Pulse	

Level of Severity	Systolic	Diastolic
Normal	120	80
Mild Hypertension	140-160	90-100
Moderate Hypertension	160-200	100-120
Severe Hypertension	Above 200	160-200

BLOOD PRESSURE LOG

NAME. ____

Date	AM		PM		Notes
	Blood pressure	Pulse	Blood pressure	Pulse	

Level of Severity	Systolic	Diastolic
Normal	120	80
Mild Hypertension	140-160	90-100
Moderate Hypertension	160-200	100-120
Severe Hypertension	Above 200	160-200

Blood Pressure Log

Name. ____

Date	AM		PM		Notes
	Blood pressure	Pulse	Blood pressure	Pulse	

Level of Severity	Systolic	Diastolic
Normal	120	80
Mild Hypertension	140-160	90-100
Moderate Hypertension	160-200	100-120
Severe Hypertension	Above 200	160-200

BLOOD PRESSURE LOG

NAME. ____

Date	AM		PM		Notes
	Blood pressure	Pulse	Blood pressure	Pulse	

Level of Severity	Systolic	Diastolic
Normal	120	80
Mild Hypertension	140-160	90-100
Moderate Hypertension	160-200	100-120
Severe Hypertension	Above 200	160-200

BLOOD PRESSURE LOG

NAME. ____

Date	AM		PM		Notes
	Blood pressure	Pulse	Blood pressure	Pulse	

Level of Severity	Systolic	Diastolic
Normal	120	80
Mild Hypertension	140-160	90-100
Moderate Hypertension	160-200	100-120
Severe Hypertension	Above 200	160-200

BLOOD PRESSURE LOG

NAME. ____

Date	AM		PM		Notes
	Blood pressure	Pulse	Blood pressure	Pulse	

Level of Severity	Systolic	Diastolic
Normal	120	80
Mild Hypertension	140-160	90-100
Moderate Hypertension	160-200	100-120
Severe Hypertension	Above 200	160-200

BLOOD PRESSURE LOG

NAME. _______________________________

Date	AM		PM		Notes
	Blood pressure	Pulse	Blood pressure	Pulse	

Level of Severity	Systolic	Diastolic
Normal	120	80
Mild Hypertension	140-160	90-100
Moderate Hypertension	160-200	100-120
Severe Hypertension	Above 200	160-200

BLOOD PRESSURE LOG

NAME. ____

Date	AM		PM		Notes
	Blood pressure	Pulse	Blood pressure	Pulse	

Level of Severity	Systolic	Diastolic
Normal	120	80
Mild Hypertension	140-160	90-100
Moderate Hypertension	160-200	100-120
Severe Hypertension	Above 200	160-200

BLOOD PRESSURE LOG

NAME. ____

Date	AM		PM		Notes
	Blood pressure	Pulse	Blood pressure	Pulse	

Level of Severity	Systolic	Diastolic
Normal	120	80
Mild Hypertension	140-160	90-100
Moderate Hypertension	160-200	100-120
Severe Hypertension	Above 200	160-200

BLOOD PRESSURE LOG

NAME. ____

Date	AM		PM		Notes
	Blood pressure	Pulse	Blood pressure	Pulse	

Level of Severity	Systolic	Diastolic
Normal	120	80
Mild Hypertension	140-160	90-100
Moderate Hypertension	160-200	100-120
Severe Hypertension	Above 200	160-200

BLOOD PRESSURE LOG

NAME. ____

Date	AM		PM		Notes
	Blood pressure	Pulse	Blood pressure	Pulse	

Level of Severity	Systolic	Diastolic
Normal	120	80
Mild Hypertension	140-160	90-100
Moderate Hypertension	160-200	100-120
Severe Hypertension	Above 200	160-200

BLOOD PRESSURE LOG

NAME. ____

Date	AM		PM		Notes
	Blood pressure	Pulse	Blood pressure	Pulse	

Level of Severity	Systolic	Diastolic
Normal	120	80
Mild Hypertension	140-160	90-100
Moderate Hypertension	160-200	100-120
Severe Hypertension	Above 200	160-200

BLOOD PRESSURE LOG

NAME. ____

Date	AM		PM		Notes
	Blood pressure	Pulse	Blood pressure	Pulse	

Level of Severity	Systolic	Diastolic
Normal	120	80
Mild Hypertension	140-160	90-100
Moderate Hypertension	160-200	100-120
Severe Hypertension	Above 200	160-200

Blood Pressure Log

NAME. ____

Date	AM		PM		Notes
	Blood pressure	Pulse	Blood pressure	Pulse	

Level of Severity	Systolic	Diastolic
Normal	120	80
Mild Hypertension	140-160	90-100
Moderate Hypertension	160-200	100-120
Severe Hypertension	Above 200	160-200

Blood Pressure Log

Name. ____

Date	AM		PM		Notes
	Blood pressure	Pulse	Blood pressure	Pulse	

Level of Severity	Systolic	Diastolic
Normal	120	80
Mild Hypertension	140-160	90-100
Moderate Hypertension	160-200	100-120
Severe Hypertension	Above 200	160-200

BLOOD PRESSURE LOG

NAME. ____

Date	AM		PM		Notes
	Blood pressure	Pulse	Blood pressure	Pulse	

Level of Severity	Systolic	Diastolic
Normal	120	80
Mild Hypertension	140-160	90-100
Moderate Hypertension	160-200	100-120
Severe Hypertension	Above 200	160-200

BLOOD PRESSURE LOG

NAME. ____

| Date | AM | | PM | | Notes |
	Blood pressure	Pulse	Blood pressure	Pulse	

Level of Severity	Systolic	Diastolic
Normal	120	80
Mild Hypertension	140-160	90-100
Moderate Hypertension	160-200	100-120
Severe Hypertension	Above 200	160-200

BLOOD PRESSURE LOG

NAME. ____

Date	AM		PM		Notes
	Blood pressure	Pulse	Blood pressure	Pulse	

Level of Severity	Systolic	Diastolic
Normal	120	80
Mild Hypertension	140-160	90-100
Moderate Hypertension	160-200	100-120
Severe Hypertension	Above 200	160-200

Blood Pressure Log

Name. ____

Date	AM		PM		Notes
	Blood pressure	Pulse	Blood pressure	Pulse	

Level of Severity	Systolic	Diastolic
Normal	120	80
Mild Hypertension	140-160	90-100
Moderate Hypertension	160-200	100-120
Severe Hypertension	Above 200	160-200

BLOOD PRESSURE LOG

NAME. ____

Date	AM		PM		Notes
	Blood pressure	Pulse	Blood pressure	Pulse	

Level of Severity	Systolic	Diastolic
Normal	120	80
Mild Hypertension	140-160	90-100
Moderate Hypertension	160-200	100-120
Severe Hypertension	Above 200	160-200

BLOOD PRESSURE LOG

NAME. ____

Date	AM		PM		Notes
	Blood pressure	Pulse	Blood pressure	Pulse	

Level of Severity	Systolic	Diastolic
Normal	120	80
Mild Hypertension	140-160	90-100
Moderate Hypertension	160-200	100-120
Severe Hypertension	Above 200	160-200

BLOOD PRESSURE LOG

NAME. ____

Date	AM		PM		Notes
	Blood pressure	Pulse	Blood pressure	Pulse	

Level of Severity	Systolic	Diastolic
Normal	120	80
Mild Hypertension	140-160	90-100
Moderate Hypertension	160-200	100-120
Severe Hypertension	Above 200	160-200

BLOOD PRESSURE LOG

NAME. ____

Date	AM		PM		Notes
	Blood pressure	Pulse	Blood pressure	Pulse	

Level of Severity	Systolic	Diastolic
Normal	120	80
Mild Hypertension	140-160	90-100
Moderate Hypertension	160-200	100-120
Severe Hypertension	Above 200	160-200

BLOOD PRESSURE LOG

NAME. ____

Date	AM		PM		Notes
	Blood pressure	Pulse	Blood pressure	Pulse	

Level of Severity	Systolic	Diastolic
Normal	120	80
Mild Hypertension	140-160	90-100
Moderate Hypertension	160-200	100-120
Severe Hypertension	Above 200	160-200

BLOOD PRESSURE LOG

NAME. ____

Date	AM		PM		Notes
	Blood pressure	Pulse	Blood pressure	Pulse	

Level of Severity	Systolic	Diastolic
Normal	120	80
Mild Hypertension	140-160	90-100
Moderate Hypertension	160-200	100-120
Severe Hypertension	Above 200	160-200

BLOOD PRESSURE LOG

NAME. ____

Date	AM		PM		Notes
	Blood pressure	Pulse	Blood pressure	Pulse	

Level of Severity	Systolic	Diastolic
Normal	120	80
Mild Hypertension	140-160	90-100
Moderate Hypertension	160-200	100-120
Severe Hypertension	Above 200	160-200

Blood Pressure Log

Name. ____

Date	AM		PM		Notes
	Blood pressure	Pulse	Blood pressure	Pulse	

Level of Severity	Systolic	Diastolic
Normal	120	80
Mild Hypertension	140-160	90-100
Moderate Hypertension	160-200	100-120
Severe Hypertension	Above 200	160-200

BLOOD PRESSURE LOG

NAME. ____

Date	AM		PM		Notes
	Blood pressure	Pulse	Blood pressure	Pulse	

Level of Severity	Systolic	Diastolic
Normal	120	80
Mild Hypertension	140-160	90-100
Moderate Hypertension	160-200	100-120
Severe Hypertension	Above 200	160-200

Blood Pressure Log

NAME. ____

Date	AM		PM		Notes
	Blood pressure	Pulse	Blood pressure	Pulse	

Level of Severity	Systolic	Diastolic
Normal	120	80
Mild Hypertension	140-160	90-100
Moderate Hypertension	160-200	100-120
Severe Hypertension	Above 200	160-200

BLOOD PRESSURE LOG

NAME. ____

Date	AM		PM		Notes
	Blood pressure	Pulse	Blood pressure	Pulse	

Level of Severity	Systolic	Diastolic
Normal	120	80
Mild Hypertension	140-160	90-100
Moderate Hypertension	160-200	100-120
Severe Hypertension	Above 200	160-200

Blood Pressure Log

Name. ____

Date	AM		PM		Notes
	Blood pressure	Pulse	Blood pressure	Pulse	

Level of Severity	Systolic	Diastolic
Normal	120	80
Mild Hypertension	140-160	90-100
Moderate Hypertension	160-200	100-120
Severe Hypertension	Above 200	160-200

BLOOD PRESSURE LOG

NAME. ____

Date	AM		PM		Notes
	Blood pressure	Pulse	Blood pressure	Pulse	

Level of Severity	Systolic	Diastolic
Normal	120	80
Mild Hypertension	140-160	90-100
Moderate Hypertension	160-200	100-120
Severe Hypertension	Above 200	160-200

BLOOD PRESSURE LOG

NAME. ____

Date	AM		PM		Notes
	Blood pressure	Pulse	Blood pressure	Pulse	

Level of Severity	Systolic	Diastolic
Normal	120	80
Mild Hypertension	140-160	90-100
Moderate Hypertension	160-200	100-120
Severe Hypertension	Above 200	160-200

BLOOD PRESSURE LOG

NAME. ____

Date	AM		PM		Notes
	Blood pressure	Pulse	Blood pressure	Pulse	

Level of Severity	Systolic	Diastolic
Normal	120	80
Mild Hypertension	140-160	90-100
Moderate Hypertension	160-200	100-120
Severe Hypertension	Above 200	160-200

BLOOD PRESSURE LOG

NAME. ____

Date	AM		PM		Notes
	Blood pressure	Pulse	Blood pressure	Pulse	

Level of Severity	Systolic	Diastolic
Normal	120	80
Mild Hypertension	140-160	90-100
Moderate Hypertension	160-200	100-120
Severe Hypertension	Above 200	160-200

BLOOD PRESSURE LOG

NAME. ____

| Date | AM | | PM | | Notes |
	Blood pressure	Pulse	Blood pressure	Pulse	

Level of Severity	Systolic	Diastolic
Normal	120	80
Mild Hypertension	140-160	90-100
Moderate Hypertension	160-200	100-120
Severe Hypertension	Above 200	160-200

BLOOD PRESSURE LOG

NAME. ____

Date	AM		PM		Notes
	Blood pressure	Pulse	Blood pressure	Pulse	

Level of Severity	Systolic	Diastolic
Normal	120	80
Mild Hypertension	140-160	90-100
Moderate Hypertension	160-200	100-120
Severe Hypertension	Above 200	160-200

BLOOD PRESSURE LOG

NAME. ____

Date	AM		PM		Notes
	Blood pressure	Pulse	Blood pressure	Pulse	

Level of Severity	Systolic	Diastolic
Normal	120	80
Mild Hypertension	140-160	90-100
Moderate Hypertension	160-200	100-120
Severe Hypertension	Above 200	160-200

Blood Pressure Log

Name. ____

Date	AM		PM		Notes
	Blood pressure	Pulse	Blood pressure	Pulse	

Level of Severity	Systolic	Diastolic
Normal	120	80
Mild Hypertension	140-160	90-100
Moderate Hypertension	160-200	100-120
Severe Hypertension	Above 200	160-200

BLOOD PRESSURE LOG

NAME. ____

Date	AM		PM		Notes
	Blood pressure	Pulse	Blood pressure	Pulse	

Level of Severity	Systolic	Diastolic
Normal	120	80
Mild Hypertension	140-160	90-100
Moderate Hypertension	160-200	100-120
Severe Hypertension	Above 200	160-200

BLOOD PRESSURE LOG

NAME. ____

Date	AM		PM		Notes
	Blood pressure	Pulse	Blood pressure	Pulse	

Level of Severity	Systolic	Diastolic
Normal	120	80
Mild Hypertension	140-160	90-100
Moderate Hypertension	160-200	100-120
Severe Hypertension	Above 200	160-200

BLOOD PRESSURE LOG

Name. ____

Date	AM		PM		Notes
	Blood pressure	Pulse	Blood pressure	Pulse	

Level of Severity	Systolic	Diastolic
Normal	120	80
Mild Hypertension	140-160	90-100
Moderate Hypertension	160-200	100-120
Severe Hypertension	Above 200	160-200

Blood Pressure Log

Name. ____

Date	AM		PM		Notes
	Blood pressure	Pulse	Blood pressure	Pulse	

Level of Severity	Systolic	Diastolic
Normal	120	80
Mild Hypertension	140-160	90-100
Moderate Hypertension	160-200	100-120
Severe Hypertension	Above 200	160-200

BLOOD PRESSURE LOG

NAME. ____

Date	AM		PM		Notes
	Blood pressure	Pulse	Blood pressure	Pulse	

Level of Severity	Systolic	Diastolic
Normal	120	80
Mild Hypertension	140-160	90-100
Moderate Hypertension	160-200	100-120
Severe Hypertension	Above 200	160-200

BLOOD PRESSURE LOG

NAME. ______________________________

Date	AM		PM		Notes
	Blood pressure	Pulse	Blood pressure	Pulse	

Level of Severity	Systolic	Diastolic
Normal	120	80
Mild Hypertension	140-160	90-100
Moderate Hypertension	160-200	100-120
Severe Hypertension	Above 200	160-200

BLOOD PRESSURE LOG

NAME. ____

Date	AM		PM		Notes
	Blood pressure	Pulse	Blood pressure	Pulse	

Level of Severity	Systolic	Diastolic
Normal	120	80
Mild Hypertension	140-160	90-100
Moderate Hypertension	160-200	100-120
Severe Hypertension	Above 200	160-200

BLOOD PRESSURE LOG

NAME. ____

Date	AM		PM		Notes
	Blood pressure	Pulse	Blood pressure	Pulse	

Level of Severity	Systolic	Diastolic
Normal	120	80
Mild Hypertension	140-160	90-100
Moderate Hypertension	160-200	100-120
Severe Hypertension	Above 200	160-200

BLOOD PRESSURE LOG

NAME. ____

Date	AM		PM		Notes
	Blood pressure	Pulse	Blood pressure	Pulse	

Level of Severity	Systolic	Diastolic
Normal	120	80
Mild Hypertension	140-160	90-100
Moderate Hypertension	160-200	100-120
Severe Hypertension	Above 200	160-200

BLOOD PRESSURE LOG

NAME. ____

Date	AM		PM		Notes
	Blood pressure	Pulse	Blood pressure	Pulse	

Level of Severity	Systolic	Diastolic
Normal	120	80
Mild Hypertension	140-160	90-100
Moderate Hypertension	160-200	100-120
Severe Hypertension	Above 200	160-200

BLOOD PRESSURE LOG

NAME. ____

Date	AM		PM		Notes
	Blood pressure	Pulse	Blood pressure	Pulse	

Level of Severity	Systolic	Diastolic
Normal	120	80
Mild Hypertension	140-160	90-100
Moderate Hypertension	160-200	100-120
Severe Hypertension	Above 200	160-200

BLOOD PRESSURE LOG

NAME. ____

Date	AM		PM		Notes
	Blood pressure	Pulse	Blood pressure	Pulse	

Level of Severity	Systolic	Diastolic
Normal	120	80
Mild Hypertension	140-160	90-100
Moderate Hypertension	160-200	100-120
Severe Hypertension	Above 200	160-200

BLOOD PRESSURE LOG

NAME. ____

Date	AM		PM		Notes
	Blood pressure	Pulse	Blood pressure	Pulse	

Level of Severity	Systolic	Diastolic
Normal	120	80
Mild Hypertension	140-160	90-100
Moderate Hypertension	160-200	100-120
Severe Hypertension	Above 200	160-200